Table of Contents

I0711404

An In-Depth Study of Acyanotic Heart Disease: Causes, Diagnosis, and Treatment

1. Introduction to Acyanotic Heart Disease

2. Epidemiology and Prevalence

23. Conclusion and Future Directions

Acyanotic Heart Disease: Types, Symptoms, Treatment, and More

1. Introduction to Acyanotic Heart Disease

Some common types of acyanotic heart disease include atrial septal defect, ventricular septal defect, coarctation of the aorta, and patent ductus arteriosus.

According to the latest statistics, acyanotic defects are more common than cyanotic defects. Moreover, many newborns live without being diagnosed with these defects. AHD describes some congenital heart defects in which the baby's blood passing through the heart and lung vessels are somehow mixed. These defects allow oxygen-poor and oxygen-rich blood to mix, even though they should not. As a result, there is a limited amount of oxygen-poor blood and a limited amount of oxygen-rich blood. These defects can occur alone or with other heart diseases.

Acyanotic heart disease (AHD) is a group of heart defects. These defects can cause structural defects in the heart that result in cardiac shunting of blood. This means the blood flow is not directed properly, resulting in the mixing of systemic and pulmonary blood. The other blood-transporting vessels may not always be in the appropriate position, not allowing enough oxygen to be transported to the rest of the body.

2. Anatomy and Physiology of the Heart

The right ventricular free wall is thinner than that of the left ventricle and has a conical shape. The ventricles are separated from one another by the interventricular septum. The left atrium receives oxygenated blood from the lungs via four pulmonary veins. It has thicker walls and a smaller volume compared with the right atrium or ventricle. Following atrial systole, the blood passes from the left atrium to the left ventricle and then, following ventricular systole, the left ventricle pumps blood around the body. During ventricular systole, the left ventricular pressure exceeds that of the aorta, leading to the aortic valve opening, and blood is ejected from the ventricle. The aortic valve closes following ventricular systole, facilitating the generation of pressure within the aorta, thereby preventing the backflow of blood into the left ventricle from the aorta.

The heart is a specialized muscle responsible for pumping blood around the body. The heart is a hollow, four-chambered organ, which is supplied with blood from the two coronary arteries on the surface of the heart. The muscle layer, or myocardium, is the layer of the heart responsible for contracting and pumping blood around the body. The chambers of the heart include the right atrium and ventricle and the left atrium and ventricle. The valves of the heart are responsible for controlling the flow of blood between the chambers, and sensitive tissue in the heart regulates the beating of the heart.

2.1. Normal Heart Circulation

The discussion of each condition is carried out in the following sequence: normal heart circulation, how a given condition alters the normal circulation, symptoms and findings based on the altered circulation, and finally, how the condition is treated. In that way, we emphasize the relationship between what is observed and heard (either through the stethoscope or by the patient's verbalization) and the altered cardiovascular physiology. We present in the initial part of the chapter the physical examination of the acyanotic child with the chief complaint of murmurs, precordial activity, and heart failure. We feel this approach will allow the reader to appreciate readily the variety of ways the acyanotic child's heart may fail to function properly and to recognize the clinical manifestations, specific findings, and natural history of his condition.

The heart of "acyanotic" children may appear normal, but for a variety of reasons, it does not function properly. The types of acyanotic heart disease are so varied that it is thoroughly classified. This chapter includes the septal defects, patent ductus arteriosus, coarctation of the aorta, and the tetralogy of Fallot. After drawing on the reader's knowledge of normal heart circulation, each condition is discussed in detail to present typical symptoms and physical examination findings. The usual treatment of each condition and the patients' short-term and long-term prognosis are also discussed.

2.2. Pathophysiology of Acyanotic Heart Disease

Acyanotic congenital heart defects (CHD) are a group of congenital defects that increase the flow of blood to the lungs and cause a left-to-right shunt. Examples of acyanotic CHD include atrial septal defect (ASD), ventricular septal defect (VSD), patent ductus arteriosus (PDA), and patent foramen ovale (PFO) with pulmonary hypertension shunt. In acyanotic congenital heart disease, there is a communication and the blood flow to the lungs increases due to the rise of pressure in the left heart. The failure of communication between pulmonary vessels and the systemic circulation results in the augmented flow to the lungs. As the flow increases, end-diastolic volume, end-systolic volume, stroke volume, and diastolic pressure of the left ventricle increase. Over time, this increases left ventricular (LV) end-diastolic volume, stroke volume, and strength. Increased pulmonary flow allows high-pressure flow, which eventually causes the crescendo-decrescendo murmur.

Acyanotic congenital heart disease (CHD) or left-to-right shunt lesions are a collection of congenital heart anomalies that increase pulmonary blood flow and eventually cause pulmonary overcirculation, increased pulmonary vascular resistance, shunt reversal, and so on. Ventricular septal defect, atrial septal defect, and patent ductus arteriosus are major examples of lesions contributing to acyanotic CHD. Persistent truncus arteriosus is a different category of left-to-right shunt lesions of acyanotic heart that causes increased pulmonary blood flow. The essential pathophysiologic theme of these defects is a deficiency in the septum creating an abnormal connection that allows a pressure gradient from a high-pressure system to a low-pressure system, causing blood to flow from left to right and increasing blood flow to pulmonary arteries.

3. Types of Acyanotic Heart Disease

The job of the right heart is to pump the blood to the lungs to receive oxygen and to get rid of carbon dioxide. There are three main obstructive lesions of the heart. These are pulmonic stenosis (PS), aortic stenosis (AS), and coarctation of the aorta (COA). The job of the left heart is to pump the blood to the rest of the body. The right heart has to work harder if it has to pump against increased resistance as in PS, AS, or COA. PS is a common heart defect. It is most often found in children, but their heart starts to hurt. It can cause breathlessness after exertion. During severe PS, a child or adult may feel faint or have a fast or irregular heartbeat. During an episode of breathlessness or fainting, the child may be heard to have a heart murmur. This sound is heard because of a small hole (defect) in the wall between the lower two heart chambers. The majority of these children have no other heart defects. They usually do not have progressive problems and will continue to grow and develop normally.

Types of acyanotic heart disease (ACD): There are two types of ACD, including high-output cardiac failure and obstructive lesions. High-output cardiac failure is a rare type of heart disease. It is often caused or brought on by chronic diseases such as anemia, beriberi, Paget's disease, and thyrotoxicosis. Other causes of high-output cardiac failure could be liver disease. In high-output cardiac failure, the body's need for blood, the amount of blood that is pumped each minute, or the volume of blood returning to the heart is too low for the amount of blood that the heart is pumping. When this happens, the heart works harder to pump more blood and the heart muscle gets even smaller and even less effective. A person may have regular or occasional symptoms for a long time before high-output cardiac failure actually develops. The person with high-output cardiac failure will usually have symptoms of heart failure. They may have normal, high, or low blood pressure. Only the heart's ability to pump is decreased.

3.1. Atrial Septal Defect (ASD)

The most common symptom of atrial septal defect is a heart murmur - a whooshing sound caused by the turbulent flow of blood. If your doctor hears a heart murmur, it may lead to a referral to a cardiologist who can help determine the cause and what treatment, if any, would be needed. In some cases, an atrial septal defect may be identified by the presence of other, more serious heart problems. A large atrial septal defect can cause extra blood to overfill the lungs and the right side of the heart. If not treated, the right side of the heart may become enlarged and fail. Over time, increased blood flow can damage the lung arteries. If the atrial septal defect is large, these extra blood flow problems can occur, and if not treated, can lead to complications.

Atrial septal defects (ASDs) are the most common congenital anomaly in adults. They're a type of atrial septal defect that occurs when the foramen ovale fails to close completely after birth. In this type, a higher than normal amount of blood flows from the left atrium to the right atrium. This usually doesn't cause any noticeable symptoms. In rare cases, a large atrial septal defect can cause shortness of breath, particularly when exercising, fatigue, swelling in the legs, feet or abdomen, heart murmurs or a stroke.

3.2. Ventricular Septal Defect (VSD)

The more blood that is shunted across a VSD, the louder a murmur generated. At a certain point, the defect gets so large that the murmur will decrease in loudness because of the damage created by the large pressure difference between the two ventricles. We know that the murmur must have been extremely loud at one time because this is the etiology of the diastolic 'rumble' murmur that a small number of otherwise normal children will generate. This murmur disappears when the defect gets large enough to equalize the ventricular pressures in diastole.

A ventricular septal defect (VSD) is a hole between the right ventricle and the left ventricle. The pressure in the left ventricle is higher than the pressure in the right ventricle. As a result, blood is shunted left to right. This means that blood that should go out the aorta is instead recirculated to the lungs to pick up more oxygen first. The body gets too much oxygen. The body eventually becomes inefficient in oxygen delivery. In fact, a VSD produces the same symptoms as coarctation of the aorta or aortic stenosis since the circulation pattern is the same.

3.3. Patent Ductus Arteriosus (PDA)

Whenever the clinical situation does not allow for immediate surgical ligation of the PDA, indomethacin can be given. Indomethacin inhibits PGE-dependent closure of the ductus arteriosus and has been effective in 80% of babies treated. Intravenously administered ibuprofen also results in PGE-dependent closure of the ductus arteriosus. During the intrauterine life of a fetus, the arterial blood from the right ventricle is shunted through the ductus into the descending aorta. The ductus arteriosus is, before birth, an essential part of the normal fetal circulation, allowing the systemic and pulmonary blood flow to remain separated. After birth, the ductus normally closes, separating the systemic and pulmonary circulations.

Patent ductus arteriosus (PDA) is a medical condition in which the ductus arteriosus fails to close after birth. Symptoms are uncommon during the first few weeks of life, although diminished blood flow to the lungs may cause breathlessness and weak 'thready' pulses. However, most small PDAs do not cause any symptoms. Severe cases present with a characteristic loud continuous machinery murmur. Patent ductus arteriosus can coexist with a number of other heart defects, including ventricular septal defect, atrial septal defect, and tetralogy of Fallot. Whether or not to treat a patent ductus arteriosus after birth has been controversial. Heart-lung machines have allowed surgical "clamping" of the PDA without stopping the heart.

3.4. Atrioventricular Canal Defect (AV Canal Defect)

The vast majority of patients with atrioventricular canal defects have associated cardiac anomalies, which can include obstruction of the left atrioventricular valve, atrioventricular valve regurgitation, ventricular septal defect requiring closure, abnormalities of the papillary muscles, presence or absence of an associated primum or secundum atrial septal defect, and associated aortic arch anomalies, as well as Shone's syndrome, truncus arteriosus, and anomalous pulmonary venous return. The malignant form is so rare that discussions in the literature show a vast difference in opinion about the name and exact components.

An atrioventricular canal defect (AV canal defect) is a combination of problems with the heart's walls, chambers, and valves. The condition is present at birth (congenital). Congenital heart disease - atrioventricular canal defect (AV canal defect); Birth defect heart - atrioventricular canal defect (AV canal defect). This defect is also commonly called an atrioventricular septal defect (AVSD). The prognosis related to atrioventricular canal defects often is determined by the severity of the associated cardiac defects. In the absence of any associated anomalies, outcomes after repair are good.

3.5. Coarctation of the Aorta

The best time to repair coarctation once diagnosed is within the baby's first few weeks of life, or better within the first few days by performing a sterile procedure to allow blood flow while limiting the hematoma and preferably leaving the ductus arteriosus open, which limits the narrowness. If the situation is not an emergency, it can also be operated on later, in a well-adjusted baby, at 6-12 months of life. In general, life expectancy is normal after surgical repair, but regular cardiovascular monitoring is recommended, especially in adulthood to detect hypertension and chronic sequelae.

Coarctation of the aorta, or coarctation for short, is a congenital malformation of the aorta. Due to coarctation, a portion of the aorta is narrow or pinched, causing the blood to flow through it more quickly and can lead to damage in the arteries involved in the blood supply. The narrowing is usually located at the point where the aorta arches near the ductus arteriosus, a blood vessel that is only open in utero and during the first weeks of life. In almost 50% of cases, this constriction is accompanied by the presence of a ductus arteriosus (a normal blood vessel that fails to close at birth). When coarctation is severe and not diagnosed early, it often leads to reduced flow to the most important arteries supplying the body, with repercussions on the development of the child and the proper functioning of the kidneys and intestines. The child may experience headaches, cold hands and feet, leg cramps and difficulty walking, and hypertension.

3.6. Pulmonary Stenosis

If caught early, treatment can help a kid recover from severe PS. The prognosis is generally good in children who get early cure. However, Parkway Hospitals can help grown-ups who get the condition treated in time escape several of the complications that PS can result in. If untreated, severe PS can result in heart issues and death in both kids and grown-ups. The best way to prevent these bad issues is to know about PS, be aware of the signs, and have it handled when signs are spotted to find a heart specialist for a test. The most recurrent cause of PS is having a dysfunctional pulmonary valve. That's frequently genetic, but can develop at random and frequently there's no family history at all. Rarely, PS can result from a muscle or artery pressing down on the pulmonary artery and stopping blood flow to the lungs. This condition's underlying cause of PS is unknown, but it is related to Turner's syndrome. Your kid's Pediatric Cardiologist will work with you to create the best course of action.

Pulmonary stenosis (PS) refers to the pathological condition where there is a narrowing of the connection between the right ventricle and the pulmonary artery. This can affect babies or children who are facing certain heart troubles. In a healthy heart, the pulmonary valve in the right ventricle directs blood flow from the heart's lower-right chamber to the pulmonary artery, which leads to the lungs. If you've been diagnosed with PS, severe constriction of PS results in the right ventricle working very hard, as it has to generate high pressure, as the muscle has to pump blood against the high resistance posed by the narrowed pulmonary valve. A selective PS can mess with your well-being at any age; however, the condition frequently can be addressed with medical care, whether you're a newborn baby or a grown-up. In infants and older children, treatment can prevent lasting damage to the new heart, so it's critical to check if your kid has the signs and receive treatment as early as they can. Kids and grown-ups who had intervention in the past and are currently symptom-free, though, have a good perspective.

3.7. Aortic Stenosis

Sometimes, findings are observed only when a child has a fever or is under stress. In some cases, the patients may experience weakness or vertigo which may also lead to sudden death. Frequent fainting is an indicator that the stenosis is severe. The symptoms will be much more significant if both mitral and aortic valves are narrowed simultaneously. Performing echocardiography helps identify aortic stenosis and an echocardiogram provides MRI-like pictures of heart. Initially, the stenosis is controlled with surgeon insertion of a catheter which ruptures the valve. The stenosis is corrected surgically by replacing the valve if the aortic stenosis does not improve as much as it is expected. Now, an "aortic stenosis valve" can be implanted which spreads when the heart is grown. No symptoms are apparent in the first 30 years after they repair.

The aortic valve prevents the aortic blood from flowing back to the left ventricle during diastole phase of cardiac cycle. Aortic stenosis is a condition, which occurs when the aortic valve or the aortic canal is narrow resulting in obstruction to the outflow of blood from the left ventricle during systole. Thus, the left ventricle has to generate very high pressure to overcome the obstruction. This condition is usually congenital and females are more commonly affected than males. The symptoms are more clearly observed at 2-3 years of age and include loss of appetite, difficulty breathing, and muscle weakness. As pressure in the systemic veins is normal, cyanosis does not occur and the systemic blood pressure is generally high. Mostly, the children with this condition are active.

3.8. Tricuspid Atresia

Surgical correction with the Fontan procedure in the neonatal period has produced survival and growth into young adulthood, although many of life's activities are limited by chronic deconditioning with decreased growth potential and low oxygen saturation, hypoxemia, and re-hypoxemia-related complications. For any significant further progress, early complete correction must allow for normal growth and continuous aerobic exercise training before the beginning of any cardiac failure and permanent heart damage.

Tricuspid atresia is a rare congenital heart disease in which the valve between the right upper chamber (right atrium) and lower chamber (right ventricle) of the heart is missing. Without this valve, blood flow from the body directly back to the lungs is impeded. The baby may have no symptoms at birth; the ductus arteriosus will have to remain patent for survival. Cyanosis is produced by an atrial septal defect or a common atrium. The lungs are likely to be damaged from the excessive pulmonary blood flow that occurs in the first days of life, following the rapid loss of prostaglandin PGE1, and the operation has to be coordinated with preoperative care following PDA closure.

4. Signs and Symptoms of Acyanotic Heart Disease

The symptoms of acyanotic lesions can look a lot like other more common heart and lung conditions as well. Because of this, acyanotic lesions can often seem like simple infections, and the underlying heart defect often isn't found.

- Trouble breathing with activities or at rest - Difficulty feeding (babies) or poor weight gain - Increased sweating - Increased rate of breathing - Frequent respiratory infections like pneumonia or bronchitis - Rapid heart rate (tachycardia) can either mean tachypnea (increased rate of breathing) or palpitations - Chest pain or dizziness in children and teenagers or fainting, especially while playing sports

If you or your child has a heart defect, you might also have symptoms. However, these symptoms can significantly depend on the affected person's age, the type, and medical condition of the heart disease, and others. Symptoms and signs of acyanotic heart disease include:

4.1. General Symptoms

Some common symptoms of acyanotic heart conditions include: - Fast breathing (tachypnea) - Higher than normal breathing rate or heart rate when resting - Rapid heartbeat - Fatigue and low energy - Slowed growth - Poor appetite - Difficulty feeding - Frequent lung infections or persistent coughing as a result of heightened lung pressures due to increased blood flow in the lungs - Exhaustion while feeding Symptoms and associated signs of congestive heart failure, e.g., tachypnea, tachycardia, swelling, increased work of breathing, diaphoresis, difficulty tolerating feeds, recurrent infections, and failure to thrive are directly related to inability to clear blood with excess volume and/or pressure from the lungs. Repeated infection and other syndromes of malaise may indicate a worsening of a previously manageable medical condition. Some less often seen symptoms are chest pain, hemoptysis, and supraclavicular neck movements.

In general, children or adults with acyanotic left-to-right heart lesions appear to be "pink" and may appear to be in no apparent distress. They may show signs of decreased exercise tolerance, diaphoresis, fatigue, tachypnea, tachycardia, irritability, and poor weight gain. In some lesions, the prominent finding may be a heart murmur, which is often asymptomatic. If the condition of the lesion results in increased blood flow from left to right (e.g., atrial septal defect), pressure from the right side of the heart increases and the patient becomes symptomatic with right-sided heart failure. Symptoms consistent with pulmonary overcirculation may be seen in total anomalous pulmonary venous return, atrioventricular septal defects, large atrial and/or ventricular septal defects, or patent ductus arteriosus. The increased work demands on the left ventricle create a left-to-right shunt, which may eventually result in irreversible pulmonary hypertension.

4.2. Specific Symptoms for Each Type

If your child's doctor suspects acyanotic heart disease, they may order several tests to make a diagnosis, including a chest X-ray, electrocardiogram, and echocardiogram. The echocardiogram is the most helpful diagnostic tool in detecting acyanotic heart defects because it shows the structure and function of the heart. According to the Children's Hospital of Philadelphia, two types of echocardiograms are commonly used: a fetal echocardiogram (performed during pregnancy) and a transthoracic echocardiogram (performed after birth).

4) Atrioventricular Canal: For kids with atrial septal defect and ventricular septal defect combined, common symptoms to look out for include feeding difficulties and a lack of growth before and after birth. Possible symptoms in a child's first year include trouble breathing, a lack of appetite, and poor weight gain.

3) Atrial Septal Defect: - Fatigue - Shortness of breath - Swelling of the legs, feet, or abdomen - Frequent respiratory infections

2) Patent Ductus Arteriosus: - Rapid breathing or shortness of breath - Difficulty feeding - Sweating with crying or during feeding - Tires easily - Swelling of the feet, legs, or abdomen - Wide pulse pressure

1) Ventricular Septal Defect: - Shortness of breath - Rapid breathing, particularly during feeding - Swelling of the feet, legs, or abdomen - Poor weight gain - Abnormal heart

rhythm - Lung damage, resulting in breathing difficulty or leading to infection

If your child has acyanotic heart disease, they may not show symptoms in the early years. If your child's doctor suspects symptoms of acyanotic heart disease after performing a physical exam, they may order a test, such as an echocardiogram, to help make a diagnosis. Acyanotic heart disease can occur alone or in combination with other heart defects. Specific symptoms depend on the particular type of acyanotic heart disease. Symptoms and associated health problems include:

5. Diagnosis of Acyanotic Heart Disease

The specific types will depend on the child's condition and situation. The following sections will provide an overview of symptoms, prognosis (common complications and if they won't be treated), prevention and suggestions, and resources for additional information on each type of acyanotic heart disease. Remember, information provided in this article is general and intended to help patients and parents become more familiar with the terms and issues associated with acyanotic congenital heart defects. These terms, medical definitions, and explanations in the provided information might also be confusing. The best practice is always to work closely with the doctor or cardiologist to help understand the situation better and discuss the treatment and management for the specific conditions.

Auscultation (listening to the patient's heart) Chest X-rays Electrocardiogram (ECG or EKG) Echocardiogram (echo) Magnetic Resonance Imaging (MRI) Cardiac catheterization (such as balloon dilation and stent placement)

In general, a variety of sophisticated tests are available to accurately diagnose the specific type of heart disease a child might have. Here are some common types of tests used to diagnose heart diseases in children:

5.1. Physical Examination

Common findings in children with heart disease, such as differential cyanosis, may not be present in the young infant. Assessment of the color should instead focus on the mucous membranes and oral mucous membranes. Systematic examination of the integument will provide clues for liver function, peripheral perfusion, and overall nutritional status. Blood pressure measurement is important to detect differences in blood pressure in the extremities, although this finding is more often seen in coarctation of the aorta beyond 2 months of age. In older children, physical examination is much less complex because greater cooperation allows for a more accurate and detailed examination. The history provided by the child can be extremely enlightening. Symptoms noted by siblings or parents are also useful. Physical activity should be at yearly intervals for recognition of late complications, such as aortic root dilation with risk for dissection and rhythm disturbances, especially atrial arrhythmias.

Evaluation for congenital heart disease should include a thorough examination of the infant, including vital signs such as pulse oximetry. Observation of breathing effort, presence and severity of dyspnea, inspection of the heart, murmurs, bruits, rate, rhythm, presence of pulses, color, temperature, and weight gain. Growth will be slowed in a severely affected older infant, but young infants may be plump unless congestive heart failure increases metabolic demands. Respiratory rate, work of breathing, and response to position changes may provide clues to the presence of heart disease. Evidence of child abuse or other non-cardiac bruises and skin color are important findings. Cyanosis can be detected, which is frequently an early sign of digital clubbing. Examination of extremities will assist in classifying the disease.

5.2. Imaging Studies

2-D color flow Doppler echocardiography is very capable of defining the size, location, functional consequences, and entire extent of the malformation. Due to its high temporal and spatial resolution, it can assess simple as well as complex anatomy very rapidly and without any significant risk to the patient of exposure to ionizing radiation. Tissue harmonic imaging enables mechanical and acoustic energy to provide a superior signal-to-noise ratio at the bubble-tissue interface and in the Doppler colored blood port, resulting in significant gains in the definition of myocardial and valvular tissue for wall motion and valve leaflet motion studies. Color flow mapping provides temporal and spatial assessment of intracardiac shunting and great arterial flow. RTPA double outlet right ventricle. Neonate with fetal history of an in-utero verified conjoined cardiac twin malformation; Intracardiac anatomy and intercardiac relationships were elaborated by IV contrast echocardiography.

FNAC classification has gained widespread acceptance as a system of categorizing congenitally malformed heart; this is a 4-tier classification (functional classification is a 6-tier system of categorizing adult congenital heart diseases) most conveniently describing congenital heart anomaly which is readily imaged during the fetal period by 4-dimensional spiral volume sonography (4D ultrasound system) and evaluated for its associated relatively severe systemic or pulmonary venous pathology [hypoplastic left ventricle syndrome and total anomalous pulmonary venous return]. Fetal echocardiography aids parental counseling, assists in patient management, and assists obstetric management by performing catheter-based intervention therapy, prenatal balloon valvuloplasty, or delivery at the appropriate time. It is essential for parents to be given enough information, comfort, and support to make an intelligent choice as they decide the next steps at this very difficult time, including whether to continue pregnancy.

Noninvasive studies provide considerable valuable information in determining the type and extent of the cardiac lesion in a child with CHD. Noninvasive echoes have superseded diagnostic cardiac catheterization in most acyanotic lesions. Accurate preoperative diagnosis and description of the location and extent of the malformation vastly decrease the need for additional invasive investigations as it helps in estimating what types and how many prosthetic grafts, patches, or conduits should be available to be used during corrective surgery. Orthotopic heart transplantation requires detailed knowledge of the anatomy of great vessels which echocardiography readily provides. A range of prenatal cardiac malformations have been diagnosed for which prenatal surgery or postnatal early intervention in the form of early balloon valvular dilation at critical aortic stenosis or early surgical correction of VSD or coarc is possible, making fetal echo or neonatal echo very valuable investigations. Optimal timing of repair can be planned by regular imaging of the heart's

function and hemodynamics by serially evaluating cardiac
anatomy.

5.3. Electrocardiogram (ECG)

Although an ECG can provide essential diagnostic information such as arrhythmias or potential coronary artery abnormalities at different ages, it may have the following limitations. The interpretation of ECG may not be accurate because of the child's age or their compensation in the early stages. A patient with volume overload can exhibit voltage changes that mimic concentric hypertrophy, which masks the true etiology. High prevalence of arrhythmias after interventions and later complications such as aortic valve regurgitation and hypertrophic cardiomyopathy in patients with ventricular septal defect.

An ECG is an important diagnostic tool used for the heart. Patients with acyanotic heart disease usually have an ECG to confirm the diagnosis. It provides information on the electrical activities of the heart. The activity is graphically traced on paper and analyzed by the physician to assess the different cardiac abnormalities for customized treatment plans. An ECG only provides information on rhythm, conduction disturbance, and certain anatomical information of the heart, ideally requiring more imaging modes to provide sufficient information. An ECG can also continuously monitor the patient's status. The incidence of some complications such as arrhythmias can be quickly detected and solved. ECG is an easy and useful tool in patients with acyanotic heart defects.

5.4. Echocardiography

Of all the diagnostic tests available, echocardiography plays the most vital role in the management of all these patients. This can be done at the bedside and it is non-invasive. Most of the tests do not require sedation. It gives the anatomical details, functional abnormalities including hemodynamic and other information about the heart. It is an excellent investigation for screening a number of patients. There is no radiation risk. The disadvantage of echocardiography is a poor acoustic window in some patients, patients with low chest (e.g. tall boys) where the beam has to travel a greater distance, and patients with lung diseases like pleural effusion or consolidation, as well as high air intensity in the chest (e.g. history of insertion of chest tube or tracheostomy). It should only be done when the information about the hemodynamics, functional and/or anatomical details of the heart is likely to affect the investigation and/or management of these patients when this information is essentially required. Normal epicardial movement and normal diameter of the ascending aorta indicate that the probability of coarctation of the aorta is unlikely. It is also used for all the NBD to assess the ventricular function in every visit and during the time when the patient is taking lots of medicine. It is also helpful in decision making and treatment of these patients. It is operator dependent.

6. Treatment Options

Treatments for heart failure, lung high blood pressure, and related problems can include the use of drugs such as ACE inhibitors, diuretics, and digoxin. A low salt diet will be recommended and, with severe cases, interests will be prompted. The outcome for people with acyanotic heart disease depends on the specific problem. Many can manage their symptoms, and others may require only careful follow-up care. In some cases, some people will require regular treatment. With careful management, several people can have an average life expectancy, meaning a life expectancy that is similar to that of a person with no heart disease.

Using a blockage in the blood vessel involves a procedure called cardiac catheterization, which can help to reduce obstructions. This is done by creating, widening, or reinforcing proper blood vessels. PDA can be treated by closing the open ductus. Opening heart surgery may be needed in some cases. This depends on the specific condition.

6.1. Medications

The most important thing that you as a parent must keep in mind is that you should never give medicines to your children that are not prescribed to them. First, discuss your child's condition with the doctor and then start giving them their proper medications.

In some other cases, doctors might have to give more medicines to the child. However, it's important to give medications to children as prescribed by the doctor and also as instructed by the pharmacist.

Furosemide: It reduces the extra water or fluid that tends to build up in the body due to heart disease. In this way, children don't feel difficulty in breathing. They can also remove the extra fluid through urination. This medicine is commonly prescribed by a pediatrician to patients with acyanotic heart disease.

Digoxin: It reduces the heart rate in children with heart failure. It also helps the heart to work well.

Medications should be given for digoxin and furosemide. These drugs include:

6.2. Surgical Procedures

The most common type of procedures rely on tubes with built-in balloons or stents. A catheter is usually a strong, hollow, flexible tube that's inserted into a vessel through the skin and can move to a narrow area. The equipment within the balloon is expanded for stretching and removal. The stent is a steel mesh. This can be balanced within the vessel to hold open the caliper. Other sorts of catheters are also often used to achieve similar objectives. Small devices with "zigzag" wire bends or strong magnets are often built into catheters. Their respective purpose is to close the connection in vessels and disable the abnormal flow of blood. Smaller heart surgery procedures can be alleviated by combined interventions. These include the ligation or clipping of small vessel connections. Small additional heart muscles are formed on veins.

Various surgical procedures can be performed in the presence of an abnormally connected vessel to redirect the flow. This may allow blood to flow to the correct vessels or away from the incorrect ones present. The intent is to decrease blood flow to the lungs. Intervention may be needed when abnormal pressure builds in the lungs due to excessive blood flow to them. Procedures may help restore balance between the body and lungs. These interventional procedures are nonsurgical except for the most complicated types.

6.3. Interventional Techniques

Introduction Cardiac catheter intervention and minimally invasive surgery are the managements of choice in many patients with congenital heart disease. In patients undergoing interventional techniques, preintervention imaging is very important. Ebstein's anomaly is not genetically transmitted, which is closely related to maternal medication, but is a sporadic disease caused by exposure during the developmental period. Nevertheless, most congenital cardiovascular diseases are multifactorial complex diseases that are closely related to genetic factors. Familial occurrence occurred in many types of heart disease, of which the proportion of offspring increases to as high as 25%. The incidence of some types of congenital heart disease is different in different regions. For example, the prevalence of ventricular septal defects (VSD) and atrial septal defects (ASD; secundum type) is unusually high in different regions. Inferring from these, some types of congenital heart disease may have a genetic background. The identification of genetic mutations will help us better understand the underlying mechanisms and provide new targets for disease diagnosis, prevention, and treatment. In recent years, with the deepening of molecular and genetic research, including hereditary factors, vascular endothelial growth factors (VEGFs), and the NRG-1/ErbB signaling pathway have complex diseases. The close relationship between heredity of growth factor signaling and the pathogenesis of congenital heart disease, this article will focus on the relationship between hereditary factors and various types of congenital heart disease that play a key role in embryogenesis.

An increasing number of patients with complex congenital heart disease now undergo catheter or hybrid interventions. A variety of procedures can reduce left-to-right shunt and pulmonary artery hypertension, and improve the quality of life in patients with atrioventricular septal defects, and develop pulmonary arteries that are stenotic or atretic. In addition to this, device closure is performed in patients without direct heart disease.

7. Prognosis and Complications

The risk of complications during pregnancy could still be influenced by various factors such as the complexity and type of cardiac defect, residual hemodynamic abnormalities, previous sternal surgery, and presence of other comorbidities. These women would need to be seen by an expert multidisciplinary team, preferably at a tertiary care center capable of managing high-risk pregnancies. They would also require discussions with the obstetrician and cardiac team, and frequent prenatal screenings with echocardiography. Among those with operative or interventional hardware, discussions would have to be held regarding potential antibiotic prophylaxis and the other risks. During labor and delivery, close cardiac monitoring and tocolysis administration, and neonatal assessment should be carried out. Often, these would be best handled in the caring hands of combined care units.

Given the different types of congenital heart diseases that exist with a variable clinical course, their natural history varies widely. The accessibility and improvement of various therapeutic modalities have increased the life expectancy of these children. The transition to an adult cardiology team would also depend on the type of congenital heart disease present, whether they underwent corrective or palliative surgery, current cardiac status, and medications being used. Most children could lead normal lives with certain restrictions on physical activity. As they grow, offspring and cardiovascular problems related to the surgery or other procedures carried out would have to be addressed and managed. Pre-conception and pre-operative counseling sessions would also have to be organized whenever indicated.

8. Lifestyle and Management Strategies

Acyanotic heart disease comprises a range of problems that affect the structure of the heart. This condition is present at birth (congenital). The blood flow between the left and right sides of the heart and between the heart and lungs is abnormally formed or blocked, making the heart work harder to properly circulate blood and oxygen throughout the body. Over time, this increased work can lead to the development of heart failure as the heart loses the ability to continue its function. Acyanotic heart disease is less severe than cyanotic heart disease. Treatment can range from observation to surgery. Common types of acyanotic heart disease include atrial septal defect (ASD), ventricular septal defect (VSD), and patent ductus arteriosus.

What You Need to Know About Acyanotic Heart Disease

Teach your child to maintain a healthy lifestyle. Teach your child about the disease, the importance of taking antibiotics to prevent infection, and to not smoke or use drugs. Closely monitor your child and take steps to recognize any potential complications.

Nothing can be done to prevent acyanotic heart disease. However, the following steps will help manage your child's condition.

9. Research and Advancements in Acyanotic Heart Disease

Although these advances and developments are moving in the right direction, for a population that has an ever-increasing prevalence, acceleration is the key. These discoveries look forward to a future improving both newborn and early diagnosis and interventions, creating a patient whose outcome is improved, in both definition and management. Two main features of acyanotic heart disease include lesser intake of oxygen through the blood and excessive pulmonary blood flow. The treatment of acyanotic heart disease is mostly managed by advanced surgeries in regards to seeing improved pulmonary blood flow in unison with effective systemic circulation flow and performance. Advanced surgery in these cases is able to correct and deliver better performance, with improvements in a specific range including subaortic chamber correction, systemic ventricle outflow tract, aortic arch obstruction or coarctation repair, unfavorable anatomy prevention, precautions taken towards residual stenosis or regurgitation, and reduction in pulmonary overflow.

Although acyanotic heart disease accounts for a large portion of congenital heart disease cases, treatment options have improved in leaps and bounds. The advance of medical equipment has allowed for diagnoses of specific tissues and cells. Advancements in areas such as 3D technologies and modeling, CCUS and MRIs, along with mobile health and medical devices make care for those dealing with many different forms of acyanotic heart disease feasible. These developments and discoveries offer advanced and better understanding of congenital heart disease, right down to the early stages of the disease genesis. Even the development of new biomaterial and advancements such as drug delivery are important in relation to treatment options.

10. Conclusion and Future Directions

Of all these patients, follow-up was the lowest in patients with small ACHDs and peripheral involvement. It is assumed that patients with small ACHDs usually do not receive proper follow-up. Regular controls of these patients are more important to prevent the development of pulmonary increased resistance and the use of operation in elder period. Additional studies are needed for this group of patients. Finally, the GROUPB study is not powered to compare the success of antifailure treatment and operation. The two groups had no control and treatment was performed entirely by the decision of the physician. Only operations that lasted for more than 120 minutes in patients who were treated medically were presented. Seven out of seven patients underwent patent ductus arteriosus embolization, and it was observed that the length of hospital stay was low. However, data on how the decision-making mechanism in all of the cases are insufficient. Future studies in this regard will carry both scientific and social empowerment.

Acyanotic heart diseases (ACHDs) are a spectrum of heart diseases with left-to-right shunt in which oxygen-rich blood is pumped back to the lungs and the body is supplied with oxygen-rich blood. In the GROUPB study, ventricular septal defect (VSD) and atrioventricular septal defect were found to be the most common ACHD types. ACHDs are usually detected early due to increased pulmonary blood flow and the symptoms of heart failure. In terms of diagnosis and follow-up, ECHO is considered the gold standard. ACHDs are mostly operated on in the two to five age range, depending on the underlying cause. Symptomatic treatment success in patients with ACHD is good. In a large number of studies, only small groups of patients with defects operated on in the neonatal and infancy period have been presented, and the desired information could not be reached. Additional studies are needed.

An In-Depth Study of Acyanotic Heart Disease: Causes, Diagnosis, and Treatment

1. Introduction to Acyanotic Heart Disease

The majority of cardiac cases in acute and emergency pediatric units were commonly identified as acyanotic heart diseases. Although these heart abnormalities sound critical and life-threatening, prompt and long-term medical care can help children from these conditions to lead a quality life. The timely study of these acyanotic heart diseases can bring remarkable change in the life of these children. In this research, we mainly focused on the causes, signs and symptoms, diagnostic methods, and the treatment options available for managing these acyanotic heart diseases. The main theme of this paper is to understand commonly seen acyanotic congenital heart diseases, the treatment available in the medical care for these children, complications, and eventually the outcome of the disease.

An in-depth study of acyanotic heart disease is vital to quickly and effectively diagnose and treat to improve the patient's quality of life. Acyanotic congenital heart disease (CHD), also referred to as the left to right shunt lesion, accounts for a significant number of patients seeking therapy from a tertiary care pediatric or adult cardiology center. Acyanotic heart diseases are characterized by mixing of arterial and venous blood which will eventually lead to Eisenmenger's syndrome. Cardiology is a branch of medical science which has faced rapid advancement and technological enhancement in recent times. Although the exact cause of acyanotic heart disease remains unknown, studies suggested that there is a strong genetic component in the development of acyanotic heart disease.

1. Introduction

2. Epidemiology and Prevalence

The prevalence of CHD varies by country and population. According to Lai et al. (2012), the Euro Heart Survey on adult CHD found a varied CHD distribution among participating European centres: some with primarily acyanotic heart disease, and others centered on complex congenital heart disease (a combination of acyanotic and cyanotic heart disease) and/or severe heart disease in ethnic minorities.

Given the tremendous fluctuation of factors that result in CHD, people born all over the world may manifest the condition. With that said, some factors can denote the likelihood of having a child with CHD. Regardless of these factors, anyone—a mother with a healthy heart or one with CHD alike—can deliver a child with CHD. This is shown by the distribution of problems noted here, such as the commonality of VSDs occurring in the general CHD population, in itself. It is influenced by the country, which is detailed in studies that detail the incidence and prevalence of CHD in different countries. Although the distribution of CHD shown here is not necessarily representative of any specific country, studies have shown various frequencies of these problems by examining different groups of people according to demographic—or country-based—classifications.

3. Embryology and Development of the Heart

The tubular heart is composed of a single, midline tube with peristaltic contractile activity, in which one non-directional contractile wave travels from the sinus venosus to the arterial pole; initially, there are no signs of separate chambers. However, at this stage, there is also an atrio-ventricular constriction. Close to the 18th day of development, cardiac septation begins to take place. The formation of the atrial or intertribal septum is characteristically formed almost simultaneously with the formation of the atrial or ventricular canals. Therefore, the formation of the intertribal septum involves the emergence of the four-chambered heart. The heart undergoes an incredibly complex process of development until it finally resembles and behaves like a fully functional, coordinated, four-chambered organ.

The embryological origin of the heart can be traced to the intraembryonic mesoderm. The development of the heart starts from a pair of endocardial tubes, which initially appear in the embryonic disc after gastrulation. These develop cranially and then fuse together with each other in an anterior-posterior direction. Subsequent early signs of heart formation, as well as the specification of mesodermal cells to become ventricular myocytes, occur early during the formation of the primitive streak and are induced by signals from the chordamesoderm. The heart begins its embryological development during the early eighth day after conception. By the third week of development, there is a cardiogenic region, and during this early growth period, the three main layers of the heart - the endocardium, myocardium, and epicardium - will begin to be formed.

4. Pathophysiology of Acyanotic Heart Disease

Acyanotic Heart Disease, as outlined in other expert systems, refers to a group of complex structural heart defects that are characterized by the presence of variable physiologic disturbances, which include abnormal heart murmurs, palpitations, arrhythmias, labored breathing, tiredness, exercise intolerance and even pulmonary hypertension at times. The condition is often associated with elevated ventricular volumes and pulmonary blood flow. Establishment of the correct diagnosis involves correlating clinical, radiographic and electrocardiographic data with findings at cardiac catheterization and angiography (using conventional cine and digital subtraction angiography, among other techniques), and both non-invasive and invasive application of RF cardiac imaging techniques. During pediatric cardiac catheterization and angiography, both oxygen saturation and hemodynamic measurements must be included in the comprehensive program to establish or exclude the diagnosis. Owing to the fact that acyanotic forms of CHD cover a broad spectrum from minor to life threatening disease, treatment of acyanotic CHD ranges from treatment over a number of years with a high likelihood of abnormal growth and normal lifespan, to immediate surgery or other intervention. In addition to the general response to CHD by the body, patient response is also determined by the underlying cause. Thus, many of the major complications linked to acyanotic CHD (including endocarditis, stroke, and decreased QoL) as well as treatment also have their origin in these causes.

Since the central cause for the impairment in individuals with acyanotic congenital heart disease (CHD) is the decreased myocardial output, the response mechanism to the decrease in blood oxygen levels evokes a compensatory elevation in heart rate. Simultaneously, a decrease in pulmonary blood flow is triggered by increased pulmonary vascular resistance (PVR) in response to reduced blood oxygen levels, whereas systemic vascular resistance (SVR) is lowered due to a decrease in systemic blood oxygen. The reduction in PVR also results in right-to-left shunting in case of a systemic-to-pulmonary collateral, therefore increasing the oxygenation of arterial blood. Moreover, a systemic-to-pulmonary collateral is usually present as well, compensating for the aforementioned decrease as it results in increased oxygenation of the arterial blood. The coexistence of a systemic-to-pulmonary collateral with a right heart volume overload, which serves as a parallel pathway, is typically investigated after age 2. This is indeed very characteristic, as it very frequently encumbers the accurate interpretation of postoperative diagnostic data. When measuring hemodynamic parameters, it is essential that the amount of shunt in flow study is corrected for that which bypasses the heart in order to properly calculate the pulmonary to systemic flow ratio and the Fick morphometry. In the presence of a coexisting collateral, this can result in an overestimation of the systemic arterial saturation.

Pathophysiology

5. Clinical Presentation and Symptoms

Severe valvar pulmonic stenosis (PS) can also present in the newborn period with cyanosis, or with cyanosis precipitated by crying, physical activity, or excitement. Most children diagnosed with acyanotic heart disease have a history of easy fatigability and rapid onset of dyspnea. A history of recurrent respiratory infections is also not unusual. A large number of causes of heart disease begin with a relatively benign period but follow a relentlessly downhill course. Therefore, it is important to recognize these conditions and bring the patients to medical attention in a timely fashion. Detection of mild cases is no less important, as moderate to severe cases have already been diagnosed clinically at an advanced stage.

Patients present with a variable clinical picture. They can be asymptomatic and come to the physician's notice incidentally during routine physical examination. The underlying diagnosis can also be detected during investigation of minor illnesses or while the child is undergoing surgery for conditions not related to the heart. Cyanosis is usually absent. Children may experience growth and developmental retardation. The symptoms or signs presented by children with this condition are usually dependent on the severity of the anomalies present, any intercurrent infections, and exposure to factors such as high altitude that may decrease pulmonary blood flow. The physical findings are very important and may suggest, to some extent, the cardiac defect underlying the patient's presentation. Some of the ominous signs include paradoxical movement of the lower chest, clubbing of the toes, ventricular enlargement, ventricular hypertrophy, and increased pulmonary viscous resistance.

Clinical presentation of patients with acyanotic congenital heart disease:

6. Diagnostic Modalities

The 'Diagnostic Modalities' section of acyanotic heart disease presents several diagnostic assessments and managements in evaluating and detecting the acyanotic defect. Both cardiac imaging and hemodynamics testing represent common diagnostic processes important in a clinical setting. Moreover, one part of the evaluation process is examining the patient's history. As a pediatric-acquired condition, the patient's underlying disease, along with other clinical manifestations, is essential in diagnostic confirmation. An important approach in examining pediatric patients for possible cardiac issues is asking about their symptoms and doing a complete physical examination. This assessment typically supplies healthcare professionals important knowledge about the likelihood of a heart defect. Currently, modern examinations and advanced diagnostic tools such as cardiac catheterization, electrocardiography, exercise testing, physical examination, and various advanced imaging methods have grown mainly in importance.

Acyanotic heart disease refers to a condition in which the heart does not have a decreased blood oxygen supply. This section describes different clinical presentations, the various defects present in acyanotic heart diseases, and their corresponding diagrams. In addition, this disease has become the main focus of pediatric acquired heart disease because it is reportedly more prevalent than the cyanotic defect. Because of many medical advancements, the survival rate of children with acyanotic heart disease has now risen. This heart condition offers a favorable development for patients; as a result, healthcare professionals find it immensely important to identify the presence of the disease as soon as possible. In this section, readers will also find information concerning the examination and assessment of the pediatric patients with a cyanotic defect, along with diagnostic studies that will aid the healthcare team in differentiating possible acyanotic from cyanotic heart defects.

7. Classification and Types of Acyanotic Heart Disease

ASD is a unique congenital heart disease requiring special focus because of its close association with left-to-right shunts and its unique clinical presentation. Here, acyanotic heart disease is classified into simple left-to-right shunts and obstruction of blood flow diseases. Simple left-to-right shunts are also classified into four subclasses of precise acyanotic heart diseases according to clinical presentation.

The Morphet classification of acyanotic heart disease is divided into eight subclasses. Class A and Class B of the Morphet classification define the heart diseases depending on pathological anatomy, with Class A belonging to diseases with decreased pulmonary blood flow and Class B including diseases with increased pulmonary blood flow. Subclasses of other classifications, like the pretruncular aortic classification and pathophysiology classification, are mentioned.

Terminology: Acyanotic heart disease, also known as left-to-right shunts or left-to-right shunting defects, is a condition of the heart with blood-to-heart shunts. In these heart diseases, oxygenated blood from one chamber of the heart (mostly the left side) flows back to the oxygenated or unoxygenated side of the heart. According to different classifications, acyanotic heart diseases are further classified into subclasses.

8. Atrial Septal Defect (ASD)

Management of atrial septal defect (ASD) is mostly symptomatic, with mild symptoms improved by medical treatment. However, surgically, either done plication patch or device closure.

The clinical presentation of ASD tends to reflect the size of the defect, the age at which complications develop, and the direction and magnitude of the resulting shunt. A large ASD can lead to volume (right heart) overload of either or both ventricles. Quiescent, "simple" septal defects and small shunts are difficult to distinguish from the normal variant with a completely occlusive "septum potential," especially if the left atrium (LA) is connected to a right ventricle. Shunt volume and echocardiography can be useful in diagnosing smaller ASD. Biochemical markers, particularly in the presence of other conduction disturbances, should be noted in patients with fifth intercostal space (ICS) parasternal systolic murmurs and/or electrocardiographic (ECG) abnormalities to exclude anomalous pulmonary venous connection secondary to an ASD.

Atrial septal defect is an anatomic defect of the atrial septum with evidence of a left-to-right shunt. The oval fossa or oval defect is in the central area of the septum secundum of the atrium. It may be isolated right ventricular volume overload and/or an enlarged right-sided chamber and valve without clinical significance enough to be called "spillage," but it is often symptomatic and causes a gradual increase in right atrial and ventricular enlargement. Rarely, patients may have fixed pulmonary increased vascular resistance leading to a change in the flow direction of the shunt, causing cyanosis.

Atrial septal defect (ASD) is an acyanotic congenital heart disease (CHD) characterized by a defect in the atrial septum, leading to left-to-right shunting of blood.

9. Ventricular Septal Defect (VSD)

There are some consequences associated with risk proportional to the RV volume overload, such as ventricular septal aneurysm, pulmonic cusp prolapse, and aortic regurgitation. Systemic embolization is a feared outcome of VSD. Early detection of VSD is required before and after birth to manage early therapeutic intervention. Ventriculography and cardiac catheterization are the gold standard diagnostic modalities. There is no gold standard treatment for VSD, however, class therapy with cardiopulmonary medication, including diuretics and vasodilators, could be sufficient to manage acute heart failure in patients with ventricular septal defects. Authoritative enlargement is not a surgery indication. Worsening of clinical symptoms with moderate exercise in ventricular septal defect with heart failure symptoms in children may not progress to correct enlargement or risk of treatment-surgery indication.

Ventricular septal defects (VSD) are a group of simple acyanotic defects with a permanent left to right shunt, causing pulmonary over-circulation and varying degrees of right ventricle (RV) enlargement. They are located in the supracristal, infundibular, trabecular, inlet, and outlet areas of the interventricular septum. RV pressure and volume overload depend not only on the size of the defect but also on the pulmonary vascular resistances. A large and unrestrictive VSD adjacent to the pulmonary valve produces further pressure overload on the pulmonary circulation. Clinical signs also depend on the size of the VSD, pulmonary hypertension, and RV volume overload to tolerate the left to right shunt in the long term. Persistence of more than 50% of systemic equalization of LV pressure in early infancy will be poor due to acute and severe pulmonary artery hypertension and congestive heart failure (CHF). If the LV pressure remains higher than systemic for more than 6 months, it will produce pulmonary artery vascular abnormality and failure to thrive. The clinical therapy approach in acyanotic CVD complicated with CHF and hemodynamic overload is divided into three phases: supportive treatment using a diuretic, cardiopulmonary medication, and therapeutic intervention. The final decision to conduct therapeutic intervention in the form of surgical or intervention closure of the VSD depends on the patient's clinical status and the size of the defect.

10. Patent Ductus Arteriosus (PDA)

PDAs are based on blood flow from the aorta to pulmonary arteries, leading to a multitude of changes in histopathology, heart, lungs, and associated blood vessels. Signs and symptoms are directly related to the size of the PDA. PDA enlargement, transluminal perforation, and pulmonary overflow are vascular pressures that cause histopathological changes. The diagnosis of PDA is based on clinical signs and confirmed by invasive and non-invasive techniques. The echo-doppler echocardiogram in the abdomen is referred to as the gold standard. The prevalence of PDAs corrected in nephroscopy and rhythm reaches 75-80 percent. The peaks of age and prevalence of PDAs increase when reaching hypothyroidism and rare diseases. Many prevalence forecasts have reported that PDA is Cole's first discovery until childhood. Although it is homozygotic in rare animals, the disease is hereditary. PDA can be increased, reduced, or complicated in time. The absence of PDA in diagnosed newborns is also called ductus arteriosus, while PDA in the undiagnosed newborn is also known as the loss of ductus arteriosus. The innocent case has been reported to be persistent for twelve weeks of age. There are other ads that regress within a few days after the newborn has been seeded. Management of PDA may include symptomatic. Indomethacin or conservative medication, computer stimulation device, medical or invasive surgical intervention, and invasive insertion surgery. However, all the interventions that exist will lead to death or severe brain injury. The preference in pharmacological prevention and management will be presented to the reader. Medical therapy can be considered or contraindicated with a Central Ductal occlusion. In English biomedical databases, SCOPUS, EMBASE, CENTRAL, PubMed-Medline, Cochrane Library, Clinical trials, and Turkish national databases will be included in a meta-analysis of studies from languages. Heterogeneity (I2 <70%) will be the effect of intellectual data, which will be performed in RevMan 5.3. With the bias ratio, considerable publication of data, small group attempts to use review studies or materials suspected of bias reporting will be used.

Patent ductus arteriosus (PDA) is a canal that connects the aorta to the pulmonary artery during fetal life and changes in the ligament after birth. PDAs are common in infancy and childhood as part of acyanotic heart disease. The clinical consequences of PDA depend on the PDA shape, size, and pulmonary vascular resistance. A large, non-restrictive PDA may result in heart failure with a predominant left or right pathology (pulmonary artery pressure exceeding half of systemic artery pressure) and/or pulmonary artery pressure. Pulmonary overflow of a continuous non-oxidizing patient is usually the first manifestation of a PDA that intervenes in infancy.

11. Atrioventricular Septal Defect (AVSD)

Atrioventricular septal defects result from deficient development of the atrioventricular canal septa. Both atrial septal and ventricular septal anomalies in these defects may vary in structure as well as in size. So, atrioventricular valve morphology is a continuum ranging from severe dysplasia to normally formed valve leaflets. A massive degree of space between the bridging leaflets of the common atrioventricular valve that protrude into the ventricles directly from the atrial level apex of the ventricular. Thus, these counter-directionally biventricular shunts are least obstructive acyanotic heart defects because of relatively equal pressure in the ventricles. Generally, they are thought to have inelastic or nearly non-compliant ventricles. Clinical presentations are generally in the second trimester with congestive heart failure in early infancy as these babies are born with ventricles infiltrated with blood (right ventricle more than left ventricle). In infancy, in case where large left-to-right shunts are present, pre-tricuspid valve regurgitation show antegrade flow reversal resulting in postductal saturation lower than ductal saturation (an indicator of marginal pulmonary vascular disease). Treatment revolves around first step creating exclusivity of this shunt between the ventricles and then correcting atrioventricular valve incompetence (if severe).

Variations in the severity of involvement may have an impact not only on management strategies and outcome prognostication but also on long-term follow-up needed for patients with acyanotic heart diseases. Anatomically, even though double inlet and balanced atrioventricular valvular connection may exist alone in the ventricular portion contributing to the anatomic substrate of hypoplastic left heart syndrome (HLHS) and straddling/overriding atrioventricular valves with displacement of a ventricular septal leaflet to the right ventricle (RV) in the absence of double-inlet left ventricle (univentricular atrioventricular connection) may precipitate a single ventricular physiology that may often show cyanosis, such defects are discussed elsewhere because of their predilection for single ventricle physiology. Specifically, atrioventricular septal defects (AVSD) have uniformly quadrifybrillar atrioventricular valvular connection, and co-exist with an additional atrioventricular connection (single) and right-to-left atrioventricular valve regurgitation to encompass the entire spectrum of AVSDs.

12. Pulmonary Stenosis

The pathophysiology of this group of anomaly is nearly always subvalvar or valvar, resistant, and progressive. Concentric stenosis can be seen with Noonan's syndrome, Alagille's disease, and in patients with congenital rubella; it can also be related to radiation therapy or to oral contraceptive hormones when patients have a history of such exposure. Symptoms—primarily exercise intolerance—are related to the severity of the obstruction rather than its cause. The most severe is seen with valvar atresia and the least severe with discrete supravalvar stenosis. Cardiac examination reveals a normal first heart sound, a right-sided loud second heart sound, a systolic ejection click after a right bundle branch block, and tricuspid regurgitation. In general, pulmonary stenosis in any form can easily be diagnosed with M-mode echocardiography. Determination of the peak gradient, the degree of stenosis, and sizing of the stenosis can be achieved with invasive arterial contraction cineangiography. Progressive pulmonary obstruction and right ventricular hypertension result in cyanosis, clubbing, and right ventricular enlargement, leading it to a more advanced form of echocardiographic and angiographic studies. Options for treatment are pulmonary balloon valvuloplasty, operative pulmonary valvulotomy, or at pulmonic stenosis, right heart bypass.

Pulmonary stenosis, a form of acyanotic heart disease, is most commonly the result of an isolated abnormality that consists of either stenosis of the pulmonary valve or, less commonly, stenosis of the branch pulmonary arteries. Obstruction can also occur both at the valvar level as well as the subvalvar or infundibular level creating concentric and eccentric forms of stenosis, respectively. Concentric stenosis may be the result of an obstructed or abnormal pulmonary valve, dysplastic or atretic pulmonary valve, pulmonary atresia or an intact ventricular septum, while the less common form of stenosis is an eccentric stenosis from causes such as a subpulmonic membrane or muscle bundle, as well as cor triatriatum dexter.

13. Aortic Stenosis

In the cardiovascular system, semilunar valves connect the ventricles with the aorta and pulmonary artery. They prevent both regurgitation (backflow of blood from the aorta or pulmonary artery into the ventricles) and stenosis (inadequate flow of blood from the ventricles into the pulmonary or systemic circulations). The aortic valve prevents backflow from the aorta to the left ventricle. The aortic leaflets are named for their anatomic orientation; the right, left coronary, and non-coronary leaflets array clockwise as viewed from the ventricular side of the leaflets. They are attached to an annular ring of connective tissue distal to the fibrous continuity between the atrial and ventricular septa.

Aortic stenosis is a type of acyanotic heart disease which accounts for 25% of all types. In this aortic stenosis, the degree of narrowing may range from mild to near/atresia. Aortic stenosis, atresia or any malformation of the aortic valve is a separate entity and has different hemodynamic behavior. In this chapter, we restrict ourselves to the study of aortic stenosis. Anatomical and Pathophysiological Study. It is very important to know the normal anatomy of the aortic valve and its clinical implications, so we must have deep knowledge about the normal and abnormal chamber anatomy where the aortic valve embeds, that is the left ventricle, aorta, and mitral valve.

14. Coarctation of the Aorta

Clinical manifestations of CoA depend on the severity of the obstruction and age of the patient. Severe CoA in the fetus often results in heart failure and intrauterine death. Newborns and neonates with CoA are usually asymptomatic apart from poor perfusion from collateral blood flow to the abdomen, pelvis, and legs. Over time, hypertension can incur myocardial remodeling which will cause heart disease. CoA is diagnosed by chest radiography and echocardiography in primary care, and in expert centers by magnetic resonance imaging, computed tomography, and cardiac catheterization. Indications for and timing of intervention in the fetus and neonate with CoA and in an older child are based on multidisciplinary discussion. CoA treatment consists of surgical or interventional repair. In the modern era of pediatrics, sophisticated diagnostic and therapeutic equipment is giving rise to a rapid increase in the burden of pediatric heart disease. Rather than trying to rely on an inappropriate adult algorithm, proper knowledge of the special regulations governing pediatric heartology for everyday clinicians is required.

Coarctation of the Aorta As another form of acyanotic CHD, coarctation of the aorta (CoA) refers to a congenital narrowing of the aorta that can be located between the branches of the left subclavian and the ductus arteriosus or below the latter in a juxtaductal position. Such stenosis impedes ascending aortic blood flow and causes a pressure gradient between the upper and lower parts of the body. Moreover, CoA enables collateral vessels to form and grow through intercostal, mammary, and abdominal vessels into a network meant to bypass the obstruction. In neonates with severe CoA, the ends of the collateral network attach directly to the pulmonary artery: this is what radiologic entities called "infantile aorta-pulmonary window" or "preductal aorta-pulmonary window". CoA is very common among people with Turner syndrome, with a prevalence of about 15-20%. CoA pathophysiology reflects the hypoplasia of the descending aorta (minimal luminal diameter less than 70% normal or less than that of the aortic valve ring) with an associated aortic isthmus of normal diameter. Thus, treatment-induced smooth reenlargement of CoA neonate will not restore the dimensions of the descending aorta.

15. Ebstein's Anomaly

Medical management: The main aim of medical therapy is to manage tricuspid regurgitation, rhythm disturbances, and heart failure. Diuretics with appropriate medical prevention should be instituted. The initial dose of diuretics must be balanced against the acceptable dose. There are many other therapies that can be offered, such as Youden-Mamzor procedures, tricuspid repair surgeries, early-onset Fontan procedure, or conversion of the late Fontan to total cavopulmonary connection. These are addressed to the supravalvar right ventricle and the tricuspid valve, if possible. They hope to increase the life expectancy of Ebstein's patients. In cases of advanced heart failure, after failing all other therapies, heart transplantation would be offerable. The presenting symptoms of an Ebstein's patient and the associated right heart failure dictate the management of the right heart disease. The tricuspid valve does not have severe anatomical defects, due to which it can be repaired as opposed to replaced. There is always the risk of post-operative need for a permanent pacemaker because of the mobile atrialized part. Residing to a life on warfarin is also feasible for otherwise healthy young patients. However, the role of these procedures and their effectiveness still are under research. Proper trials should be carried out before becoming the routine management of an Ebstein's anomaly.

Presentation: The clinical manifestation is varied among patients. Typically, there are: (i) right atrial enlargement; (ii) atrialization of a part or the whole of the right ventricle that can pose a diagnostic problem for the sonographer; (iii) displacement and stenosis of the tricuspid valve that give rise to all degrees of tricuspid regurgitation; and (iv) varying amounts of overriding of the orifice of the tricuspid valve that leads to the atrialized right ventricle. The ECG shows diffuse T-wave inversion and current of injury in the right precordial leads. Finally, hepatomegaly is present (i.e., "hepatojugular reflux"), which can show the functional right ventricular performance. Diagnosing an Ebstein's anomaly confirms the genetic defect, which may have inter-familial consequences.

Ebstein's anomaly is a specific and rare form of abnormally downward apical displacement of the site of septal leaflet of the tricuspid valve. Anomalies are not just limited to the tricuspid leaflets but are coupled with a variable amount of right ventricular dilation. In addition, there are other structural and functional right ventricular anomalies and associated cardiac malformations. There are three important typical features of Ebstein's anomaly: (i) adhesion and abnormal tricuspid valve septal leaflet that shifts below the valvular body ring; (ii) in approximately 90% of cases, accessory and septal leaflets of the tricuspid valve are fused into a 'common atrioventricular valve'. If they are not completely fused, they still are hyperplastic; and (iii) Supra-valvular obstruction to the right ventricle by the displacement of the tricuspid valve leaflets.

16. Management and Treatment Options

A multifaceted approach is often used to manage patients with acyanotic heart disease, even though they often remain asymptomatic for extended periods of time. Gene therapy and stem cell therapy are two emerging treatment modalities. The disease often necessitates the use of catheter-based or surgical repair techniques. The aim of treatment in such patients is to improve systemic ventricular function, address valvar regurgitation and stenosis, and reduce outflow obstruction. In some cases, the disease is associated with the development of arrhythmias, which could necessitate the use of anti-arrhythmic medications or a major procedure called catheter ablation, which consists of the removal of the tissues in charge of causing an abnormal rhythm.

The management of acyanotic heart disease begins with therapeutic strategies tailored specifically for the patient. Patients can present with or without symptoms, depending on the cardiac anatomy present and its associated blood flow pattern. Some of these interventions are medical and focus on minimizing symptoms, while others are surgical or interventional procedures designed to correct or improve the underlying issue. Both medical and surgical interventions are aimed at normalizing the patient's hemodynamics to prolong life expectancy, reduce associated morbidities and hospital admissions, as well as to avoid unnecessary hospital admissions and, in some cases, the premature onset of complications.

17. Medical Management

suggested that lifestyle modification for children with CHD included maintenance of dental hygiene, limitation of salt intake by focusing on a high-potassium food diet rather than salt restriction, maintenance of an adequate level of physical activity, avoidance of weight gain and dehydration, and avoidance of isometric exercise. Ongoing monitoring for chronic complications is recommended for these patients. Macrophage motility is the most common cause of death. Thus, diagnosis and treatment are necessary, particularly in eastern Sudan, where the delta reaches 12.4 deaths per 100,000. In this study, we investigated the effect of medical and surgical treatment on patients with acyanotic heart disease.

The aim of the pharmacological approach is to manage symptoms, optimize cardiac function, and prevent arrhythmias, bacterial endocarditis, blood clot formation, and heart failure. The pharmacological management of acyanotic heart defects includes the treatment of tachycardia, heart failure, and arrhythmias; low-dose aspirin administration for adequate prophylaxis against infective endocarditis; diuretics for the treatment of symptoms of heart failure such as congestive cardiac failure and pericardial effusion; and antiarrhythmics. Pacing is used for patients with conduction disease and sinus node dysfunction, presupposing an appropriate standard in the United States for symptomatic patients with acquired complete heart block and a class I recommendation for patients with acquired advanced or second-degree atrioventricular (AV) block.

18. Surgical Interventions

The Blalock-Taussig shunt for increasing the size of the pulmonary artery increases the amount of blood sent to the lung while it does not cure the cause of higher pressure in the pulmonary circulation. Surgery uniquely designed for a unique cardiac disease may be too time-consuming or is not always technically possible. In that situation, a surgeon may perform palliative surgery as a first or interim step directed toward increasing blood flow to the lungs and plan for the definitive procedure later. The principal advantage of a palliation is that surgery can be performed quickly, possibly through a minimally invasive technique (catheterisation technique in some cases). Palliative surgery can be, in some exceptional cases, also performed in newborns with severe co-morbidities, preventing a major reconstructive surgery.

Surgical intervention is, in conjunction with medical therapy, an important aspect of acyanotic heart defect management. The principal indications for surgery in acyanotic heart diseases include the correction of obstructive valvar and subvalvar anomalies, correction of abnormal vessel connection and related anomalies to provide anatomical correction. Complete relief of valvar and subvalvar stenosis and regurgitation may be needed to improve ventricular function. Surgical intervention may aim at increasing blood flow to the heart muscle or overcome the abnormalities, which restrict physical activity and prevent cardiovascular symptoms. It can be directed towards the correction of anatomical anomalies, such as valve repair, closure of defects and excision of muscle bundles, leading to obstructed blood flow through the heart. The surgery can result in the restoration of normal circulatory connections, such as the arterial switch for transposition of great arteries, Senning or Mustard operation for the transposed arteries.

19. Interventional Cardiology Procedures

Additionally, the expansion of interventional cardiology combined with surgical rectification is a novel strategy. However, it remains an experimental preliminary and perhaps appears not yet completely effective. The ability of interventional cardiology therapies is continuously enhancing to enable more and more dealing interest in acyanotic heart disease. Development in the advance of novel tools for treatment of the heart cannot ignore to review in the same way the adult approach of patients with congenital heart defects. Noteworthily, mainly in pediatric cases in the entire world, the results of the plentiful available data may enhance the enrollment in the congenital intervention led by the different adult-derived structure. In detail, the translational openings are starting to regard the technically effective and surgically ineffective revivals.

Interventional cardiology procedures are carried out for various acyanotic heart diseases. These interventions can generally be new innovations involving new technologies, original pediatric expertise, or conservative adult technological approaches. The portfolio includes a variety of catheter-based miniaturized techniques as well as alternative minimally invasive surgery, with which distinct cardiac morphological features can be treated. Frequently, residual pediatric cardiological therapeutic approaches now accompany and possibly avoid surgery in alternative transcatheter interventions. These procedures are especially invaluable in congenital heart disease, where most but not all children are primarily treated, especially if the defect cannot necessarily be closed or thermalized. It may play a complimentary role in the recent practice of different sub-disciplines, particularly adult congenital heart disease, pediatric cardiology, and even less frequently in the fetal field.

20. Long-Term Prognosis and Complications

Patients who have moderate to severe left to right shunting across an intracardiac connection (Three's a crowd: ASD, VSD, PDA) or significant valvar stenosis face an increased risk of developing Eisenmenger syndrome. For patients with persistent significant intracardiac right to left shunting or left heart obstructive lesions requiring medication or surgery, the risk of ventricular dysfunction and the need for palliative care exists as well. In general, the opening or closing of intracardiac connections, relief of intracardiac obstructions, and provision of relief from valvar stenosis should in most cases provide the affected patient with freedom from their congenital heart condition and resume normal daily living. Patients may have a decreased exercise capacity, and the presence of pulmonary hypertension may make normal day to day activities like walking or sports uncomfortable, but these patients may not typically expect a shortened life expectancy.

A variety of factors impact the prognosis for patients with acyanotic congenital heart disease. The anatomic malformations that are the primary defect represent a broad spectrum of potential outcomes in terms of the overall diagnosis, associated findings, and long-term outcomes. Patients who have surgical repair of coarctation of the aorta and an otherwise normal heart should have a normal or nearly normal life expectancy, free from heart-related restriction. While patients who have an atrial septal defect or a ventricular septal defect repaired may have mildly decreased exercise capacity and residual restrictions to activity, these patients should also generally expect normal or nearly normal lifespans. In patients who have aortic stenosis, the peak velocity of left ventricular ejection (measured in m/sec) as determined by echocardiogram or cardiac MRI is considered to be the most important in predicting which children will require intervention, be it open-heart surgery or balloon dilation.

21. Pregnancy and Acyanotic Heart Disease

For any woman of reproductive age, it is helpful for the family planning consultation to provide information regarding the risks associated with pregnancy alongside advice on the most appropriate forms of contraception. This is particularly pertinent to women with cardiac disease who may be at increased risk of adverse maternal and fetal outcomes. Accordingly, it should be reinforced that pregnancy in women with acyanotic heart disease is generally well tolerated, with the greater part of these women mothering successful outcomes. Pregnancy should therefore not automatically be discouraged, and it is paramount that this is discussed openly with women, particularly as there is evidence to suggest pregnancy is declining in many women with adult congenital heart disease. Careful counseling by an adult congenital heart disease multidisciplinary pregnancy team should help women make an informed decision regarding pregnancy. Maternal demands of pregnancy alongside normal physiological adaptations experienced will be pertinent moving forward, but importantly, concerns regarding pregnancy should include both maternal and fetal well-being, a concept known as two-patient obstetrics.

Pregnancy is generally well-tolerated in individuals with an acyanotic cardiac lesion. However, the cavopulmonary connection group of complex lesions, in which the pulmonary circulation is dependent on passive flow from the systemic veins, have long-term implications affecting maternal and fetal health including failure of the single ventricle and fetal growth restriction. The care of these women is complex and should involve joint obstetric and cardiac multidisciplinary teams, and the provision of up-to-date epidemiology data will facilitate this.

22. Research and Advances in the Field

Clinical trials: A study will begin by invitation. Twenty-five pregnant women who have had the prenatal examination to confirm that there is a ventricular septal defect alone will be re-examined using detailed echocardiography in the first few days after delivery to confirm the absence of an ASD. Only those with a ventricular septal defect alone will be asked to participate in the trial. Because this study aims to identify the effect of adding Digoxin to the standard current treatment option of increased oral fluid, the trial will enroll those infants unlikely to need the use of the generic drug Sildenafil. Randomization will then be with or without the addition of 7 days of Digoxin therapy. The dose will be based on studies completed in India, which have been congruent with a controlled study of European and American infants. Currently, no research has been published about the management of severe symptoms in these babies. If the addition of Digoxin proves effective, it will provide strong incentive for this therapy to be more broadly used and included in the larger version of the trial. Given the severity of the condition, it is very unlikely in these babies that there will be any adverse effects associated with the use of Digoxin. In addition to benefits seen at the trial endpoint of 28 days, this will be of longer benefit by also preventing injury to the lung vessels, and potentially avoiding the longer-term need for invasive procedures such as cardiac catheterization and guiding the use of medicine. Long-term follow-up studies will determine whether these medications provide any longer-term benefits.

Experimental study: Low-magnitude mechanical stimuli (LMMS) have been reported to enhance proliferation of multiple cell types as well as to increase ECM generation, making LMMS a promising therapeutic. While the exact mechanism or mechanisms behind the biological responses to LMMS are not yet fully understood, it has been demonstrated in vitro and in vivo that LMMS leads to ERK1/2 phosphorylation in a number of different cells, including cardiac fibroblasts. The development of novel array-based technologies, such as transcriptomics and proteomics, has allowed for simultaneous examination of many different genes and proteins on a single chip. Using these powerful new tools, we chose to examine the combined effects of mechanical stimuli on gene and protein expression. This study is the first to examine in a detailed manner the intracellular changes involved in mechanical conditioning in the heart, more specifically through the increased understanding of how and when mechanical signals are converted into changes in gene expression, in particular, BNP, in cardiac fibroblasts. More detailed exploration of the cellular changes will involve array-based technologies to establish the mechanisms by which cells respond to external stimuli and modulate their role in tissue repair and disease progression.

New technologies and methods: With the development of ultrasound equipment and improvement of the operational level, the diagnosis of heart disease has made great progress in recent years. Real-time Color Doppler Flow Imaging (CDFI) echocardiography has become a main method for the diagnosis of heart disease. Besides providing two-dimensional images of the heart structure, CDFI also achieves a special simultaneous display of two-dimensional images and hemodynamic changes, by observing the color of blood flow in the heart and vessels with CDFI. This function makes the clinical diagnosis and dynamic observation of congenital heart disease much easier and more credible.

23. Conclusion and Future Directions

In utero and postnatal, if heart surgery or catheter treatment is needed, should be treated in time. In severe cases, early heart surgery is needed to correct the cause of the disease. For mild cases, only regular follow-up and observation are required. In utero, if severe heart failure develops or other important organs are damaged, such as liver and kidney damage, the risk of perinatal death increases and timely termination of pregnancy should be considered. Finally, some rather sophisticated technologies, such as genetic mosaicism, single-cell sequencing, and transcriptome sequencing, should not be ignored but used extensively as they can provide novel and valuable perspectives for future exploration of acyanotic heart diseases.

Acd, a subclass of congenital heart disease, is common in clinical practice. Through the study, we found that the pathogenesis of acd was relatively complex and not fully deciphered, being related to genes, teratogenicity, and immune factors. Even though the results suggest the potential of genetic mutation, and a clinical path for the diagnosis and relevant treatment, such as a tumor or immune-related cotrehcp, has been identified. The challenge, however, is that the gene mutation analysis, the major method for acd diagnosis, is limited owing to high price and low accuracy mainly due to genetic heterogeneity. With the development of technology, genetic mosaicism, single-cell sequencing, and transcriptome sequencing can be used to further analyze the genetic and immune factors involved in acyanotic congenital heart disease.

www.ingramcontent.com/pod-product-compliance
Lightning Source LLC
Chambersburg PA
CBHW070750250726
48662CB00004B/1729